Depression
WHERE

JOURNAL TO RECOVERY

BRIANA ISHAM

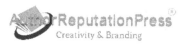
AuthorReputationPress®
Creativity & Branding

Cover Designer: Francis B.

Briana Isham
Visit my website at www.composedartistry.com

Author Reputation Press LLC
45 Dan Road Suite 36
Canton MA 02021
www.authorreputationpress.com
Hotline: 1(800) 220-7660
Fax: 1(855) 752-6001

Ordering Information:
Quantity sales. Special discounts are available on quantity purchases by corporations, associations, and others. For details, contact the publisher at the address above.

Printed in the United States of America.

ISBN-13: Softcover 978-1-952250-22-4
eBook 978-1-952250-23-1

Library of Congress Control Number: 2020904926

I wanted to talk about it. Damn it. I wanted to scream. I wanted to yell. I wanted to shout about it. But all I could do was whisper "I'm fine."

—Briana Isham

This journal is dedicated to all men, women, and children that need help. Those who don't know where to turn, or who they can trust. Sometimes you want to scream to the heavens, but no one hears your cries. They say this world is becoming sensitive when the world is becoming evil. Can you imagine your child hurting so bad and you never knew what was wrong or even that there was a problem? This journal is to help these individuals help those around and even themselves see that there is a problem, and this is their scream!!!!!!

LIST OF PROFESSIONALS

<u>National Suicide Prevention Lifeline</u>
Call 1-800-273-8255

Youth Hotlines

The above crisis hotline is available for both adults and youths. If you're looking for a youth-specific line, you can try one of the following:

- <u>Trevor Project Lifeline</u> – Hotline for LGBT youth
  866-488-7386

- <u>Child Help USA National Hotline </u>– For youth who are suffering from child abuse
  1-800-4-A-CHILD (1-800-422-4453)

- <u>Boys Town National Hotline</u> – Serving all at-risk teens and children
  800-448-3000

- <u>National Teen Dating Violence Hotline </u>– Concerns about dating relationships
  1-866-331-9474 or text "loveis" to 22522

DEPRESSIVE SYMPTOMS

- Depressed mood most of the day, nearly every day, as indicated by either subjective report (e.g., feeling sad, blue, "down in the dumps," or empty) or observations made by others (e.g., appears tearful or about to cry). (In children and adolescents, this may present as an irritable or cranky, rather than sad, mood.)
- Markedly diminished interest or pleasure in all, or almost all, activities every day, such as no interest in hobbies, sports, or other things the person used to enjoy doing
- Significant weight loss when not dieting or weight gain (e.g., a change of more than 5 percent of body weight in a month), or decrease or increase in appetite nearly every day
- Insomnia (inability to get to sleep or difficulty staying asleep) or hypersomnia (sleeping too much) nearly every day
- More days than not, problems with sitting still, including constant restlessness, pacing, or picking at one's clothes (called *psychomotor agitation* by professionals); or the opposite, a slowing of one's movements, talking very quietly with slowed speech (called *psychomotor retardation* by professionals)
- Fatigue, tiredness, or loss of energy nearly every day — even the smallest tasks, like dressing or washing, seem difficult to do and take longer than usual
- Feelings of worthlessness or excessive or inappropriate guilt nearly every day (e.g., ruminating over minor past failings)
- Diminished ability to think or concentrate, or indecisiveness, nearly every day (e.g., appears easily distracted, complains of memory difficulties)
- Recurrent thoughts of death (not just fear of dying), recurrent suicidal ideas without a specific plan, or a suicide attempt or a specific plan for committing suicide

DEPRESSION TEST

If most of your answers are between Just a little, Somewhat, Moderately, quite a lot, very much you may want to consult with a professional:

1. I do things slowly.
    Not at all
    Just a little
    Somewhat
    Moderately
    Quite a lot
    Very much

2. My future seems hopeless.
    Not at all
    Just a little
    Somewhat
    Moderately
    Quite a lot
    Very much

3. It is hard for me to concentrate on reading.
    Not at all
    Just a little
    Somewhat
    Moderately
    Quite a lot
    Very much

4. The pleasure and joy have gone out of my life.
    Not at all
    Just a little
    Somewhat
    Moderately
    Quite a lot
    Very much

5. I have difficulty making decisions.
    Not at all
    Just a little
    Somewhat
    Moderately
    Quite a lot
    Very much

6. I have lost interest in aspects of life that used to be important to me.
    Not at all
    Just a little
    Somewhat
    Moderately

Quite a lot

Very much

7. I feel sad, blue, and unhappy.

Not at all

Just a little

Somewhat

Moderately

Quite a lot

Very much

8. I am agitated and keep moving around.

Not at all

Just a little

Somewhat

Moderately

Quite a lot

Very much

9. I feel fatigued.

Not at all

Just a little

Somewhat

Moderately

Quite a lot

Very much

10. It takes great effort for me to do simple things.

Not at all

Just a little

Somewhat

Moderately

Quite a lot

Very much

11. I feel that I am a guilty person who deserves to be punished.

Not at all

Just a little

Somewhat

Moderately

Quite a lot

Very much

12. I feel like a failure.

Not at all

Just a little

Somewhat

Moderately

Quite a lot

Very much

13. I feel lifeless—more dead than alive.

Not at all

Just a little

Somewhat

Moderately

Quite a lot

Very much

14. My sleep has been disturbed—too little, too much, or broken sleep.

Not at all
Just a little
Somewhat
Moderately
Quite a lot
Very much

15. I spend time thinking about HOW I might kill myself.

Not at all
Just a little
Somewhat
Moderately
Quite a lot
Very much

16. I feel trapped or caught.

Not at all
Just a little
Somewhat
Moderately
Quite a lot
Very much

17. I feel depressed even when good things happen to me.

Not at all
Just a little
Somewhat
Moderately
Quite a lot
Very much

18. Without trying to diet, I have lost, or gained, weight.

Not at all
Just a little
Somewhat
Moderately
Quite a lot
Very much

Discovering How the Darkness Formed

WHERE ARE YOU?

Depression is classified as a mood disorder. It may be described as feelings of sadness, loss, or anger that interfere with everyday activities.

Here is where you may test some symptoms you may be having......

- weight gain or loss

- physical pain

- substance use problems

- emotional roller-coaster

- panic attacks

- relationship problems

- social isolation

- suicidal thoughts

- self-mutilation

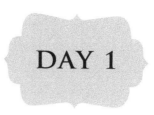

DAY 1

How was your day today?

_____

_____

_____

_____

_____

_____

_____

_____

_____

_____

_____

_____

_____

_____

_____

_____

_____

_____

_____

_____

_____

_____

_____

_____

_____

_____

HOW CAN YOU HAVE A GREAT DAY TOMORROW?

You may say that is a hard question to answer but let's think how did you overcome yesterday?

- Did you speak with friends?

- Did you speak to your family?

- Did you think of happy thoughts?

- Did you do something that makes you happy?

- Do you have a hobby? If yes, what is it?

- Did you buy something that makes you smile?

_____

_____

_____

_____

_____

_____

_____

_____

_____

_____

_____

_____

_____

Sometimes we fall but don't let that fall stop your success to greater things pick yourself up and dust off. Sometimes we have to fall once so we won't fall again.

–Briana Isham

Depression doesn't go away overnight. it's a process you must work through within to see and better horizon.

- It's the little things that help throughout the day.

- It's someone making you smile.

- It's seeing your favorite pet.

- It is seeing the people who love you.

- Its knowing that you are loved.

- Its knowing that all dark moments don't last forever.

- It's knowing that it's okay to cry.

- Its knowing that it's okay to be sensitive.

_____

_____

_____

_____

_____

_____

_____

_____

_____

_____

_____

_____

_____

_____

"There is hope, even when your brain tells you there isn't."

—John Green

DAY 2

How was your day today?

_____
_____
_____
_____
_____
_____
_____
_____
_____
_____
_____
_____
_____
_____
_____
_____
_____
_____
_____
_____
_____
_____

HOW CAN YOU HAVE A GREAT DAY TOMORROW?

You may say that is a hard question to answer but let's think how did you overcome yesterday?

- Did you speak with friends?

- Did you speak to your family?

- Did you think of happy thoughts?

- Did you do something that makes you happy?

- Do you have a hobby? If yes, what is it?

- Did you buy something that makes you smile?

_____

_____

_____

_____

_____

_____

_____

_____

_____

_____

_____

_____

_____

_____

What depression is really like:

- not showering regularly

- not brushing your teeth regularly

- living in filth

- caring about grades but not enough to do anything about them

- thinking about suicide more than graduating

- considering suicide whenever any problem arises

- tired

- no motivated

- no energy

- walking is so hard

- sometimes even talking is too much work because you're so damn tired

- lying in bed for hours because you're too tired to move

- feeling nothing but sometimes everything

- knowing you're not alone but still feeling alone

- that constant mindset of, "who cares? I won't be around much longer anyway."

Do you hate when people say it's all in your head, get over it? Think positive, get out and do things?

If that answer is yes, then here's what to say back......

Back Off!!!!

Then count to 10 and say listen I hear you I understand you, but you need to understand me. I am taking this a day at a time, I am trying to stay out of dark clouds in my head and you sir or ma'am are not making it easier for me to do that by saying your ignorant rants to me about how the freak I feel inside. Now if you would kindly back the bakeoff or help me get better, I will see your negativity out of the door.

Thank you kindly!!!!!!

I have endured pain and loss, I have felt broken, I have known hardship, and I have felt lost and alone.

But here I stand, trying to move forward, one day at a time. I will remember the lessons in my life because they are making me who I am.

Stronger.

—A warrior

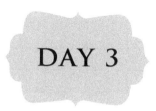

DAY 3

How was your day today?

_____

_____

_____

_____

_____

_____

_____

_____

_____

_____

_____

_____

_____

_____

_____

_____

_____

_____

_____

_____

_____

_____

_____

_____

_____

_____

_____

_____

HOW CAN YOU HAVE A GREAT DAY TOMORROW?

You may say that is a hard question to answer but let's think how did you overcome yesterday?

- Did you speak with friends?

- Did you speak to your family?

- Did you think of happy thoughts?

- Did you do something that makes you happy?

- Do you have a hobby? If yes, what is it?

- Did you buy something that makes you smile?

_____

_____

_____

_____

_____

_____

_____

_____

_____

_____

_____

_____

_____

_____

"Laughter and Tears are both responses to frustration and exhaustion. I myself prefer to laugh, since there is less cleaning up to do afterward."

–Kurt Vonnegut

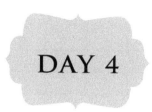

DAY 4

How was your day today?

_____
_____
_____
_____
_____
_____
_____
_____
_____
_____
_____
_____
_____
_____
_____
_____
_____
_____
_____
_____
_____
_____
_____
_____
_____
_____
_____

HOW CAN YOU HAVE A GREAT DAY TOMORROW?

You may say that is a hard question to answer but let's think how did you overcome yesterday?

- Did you speak with friends?

- Did you speak to your family?

- Did you think of happy thoughts?

- Did you do something that makes you happy?

- Do you have a hobby? If yes, what is it?

- Did you buy something that makes you smile?

You look happy, but you don't feel happy. That's what depression does to you.

–Unknown

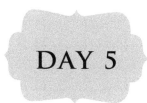

DAY 5

How was your day today?

_____
_____
_____
_____
_____
_____
_____
_____
_____
_____
_____
_____
_____
_____
_____
_____
_____
_____
_____
_____
_____
_____
_____
_____
_____
_____
_____
_____
_____
_____

HOW CAN YOU HAVE A GREAT DAY TOMORROW?

You may say that is a hard question to answer but let's think how did you overcome yesterday?

- Did you speak with friends?

- Did you speak to your family?

- Did you think of happy thoughts?

- Did you do something that makes you happy?

- Do you have a hobby? If yes, what is it?

- Did you buy something that makes you smile?

_____
_____
_____
_____
_____
_____
_____
_____
_____
_____
_____
_____
_____
_____
_____

People think depression is sadness. People think depression is crying. People think depression is dressing in black. But people are wrong. Depression is a constant feeling of being numb. Being numb to emotions, being numb to life. You wake up in the morning just to go back to bed again.

Starting to Heal

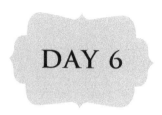

DAY 6

How was your day today?

Living- the pursuit of a lifestyle of the specified type.

Existing- is used to describe something which is now present, available, or in operation, especially when you are contrasting it with something which is planned.

Which are you doing living or existing?

_____

_____

_____

_____

_____

_____

_____

_____

_____

_____

_____

_____

_____

_____

_____

_____

_____

_____

_____

_____

HOW CAN YOU HAVE A GREAT DAY TOMORROW?

You may say that is a hard question to answer but let's think how did you overcome yesterday?

- Did you speak with friends?

- Did you speak to your family?

- Did you think of happy thoughts?

- Did you do something that makes you happy?

- Do you have a hobby? If yes, what is it?

- Did you buy something that makes you smile?

_____

_____

_____

_____

_____

_____

_____

_____

_____

_____

_____

_____

_____

_____

On particularly rough days when I'm sure I can't possibly endure, I like to remind myself that my track record for getting through bad days so far, is 100% and that's pretty good.

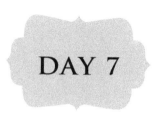

DAY 7

How was your day today?

_____

_____

_____

_____

_____

_____

_____

_____

_____

_____

_____

_____

_____

_____

_____

_____

_____

_____

_____

_____

_____

_____

_____

_____

_____

_____

HOW CAN YOU HAVE A GREAT DAY TOMORROW?

You may say that is a hard question to answer but let's think how did you overcome yesterday?

- Did you speak with friends?

- Did you speak to your family?

- Did you think of happy thoughts?

- Did you do something that makes you happy?

- Do you have a hobby? If yes, what is it?

- Did you buy something that makes you smile?

_____

_____

_____

_____

_____

_____

_____

_____

_____

_____

_____

_____

_____

_____

_____

_____

What could you do to move your energy to something that makes you happy?

Some examples are:

- basketball
- baseball
- running
- exercising
- art
- poetry
- rapping
- writing
- reading
- going out

come up with your own list of things that make you happy.......

_____

_____

_____

_____

_____

_____

_____

_____

_____

_____

_____

_____

_____

_____

YOUR LIST HERE:

_____
_____
_____
_____
_____
_____
_____
_____
_____
_____
_____
_____
_____
_____
_____
_____
_____
_____
_____
_____
_____
_____
_____
_____
_____
_____
_____

Give yourself another day, another chance. You will find your courage eventually. Don't give up on yourself.

–Unkwon

DAY 8

How was your day today?

_____
_____
_____
_____
_____
_____
_____
_____
_____
_____
_____
_____
_____
_____
_____
_____
_____
_____
_____
_____
_____
_____
_____
_____

HOW CAN YOU HAVE A GREAT DAY TOMORROW?

You may say that is a hard question to answer but let's think how did you overcome yesterday?

- Did you speak with friends?

- Did you speak to your family?

- Did you think of happy thoughts?

- Did you do something that makes you happy?

- Do you have a hobby? If yes, what is it?

- Did you buy something that makes you smile?

_____

_____

_____

_____

_____

_____

_____

_____

_____

_____

_____

_____

_____

Draw a picture of your happiest moment and share it to me on Instagram: @composedartistry or Facebook: @ComposedArtistry

DAY 9

How was your day today?

_____

_____

_____

_____

_____

_____

_____

_____

_____

_____

_____

_____

_____

_____

_____

_____

_____

_____

_____

_____

_____

_____

_____

_____

_____

_____

_____

HOW CAN YOU HAVE A GREAT DAY TOMORROW?

You may say that is a hard question to answer but let's think how did you overcome yesterday?

- Did you speak with friends?

- Did you speak to your family?

- Did you think of happy thoughts?

- Did you do something that makes you happy?

- Do you have a hobby? If yes, what is it?

- Did you buy something that makes you smile?

_____

_____

_____

_____

_____

_____

_____

_____

_____

_____

_____

_____

_____

_____

When you feel as though you don't want to get out of bed, what is happening when you feel that way?

Let's write down some affirmations you can remember to say every morning.

Here are some examples:

- I am worthy

- I am enough

- I am beautiful

- I am handsome

- I am intelligent

- I can do anything

_____

_____

_____

_____

_____

_____

_____

_____

_____

_____

_____

_____

_____

_____

_____

_____

_____

_____

YOUR LIST CONTINUED:

Having anxiety and depression is like being scared and tired at the same time. It's the fear of failure, but no urge to be productive. It's wanting friends but hates socializing. It's wanting to be alone, but not wanting to be lonely. It's feeling everything at once then feeling paralyzingly numb.

–Unkown

A manifestation which means an event, action, or object that clearly shows or embodies something, especially a theory or an abstract idea.

Exercise:

I want you to **practice or experiment with visualization of what you manifest:**

1. Think about what you want to manifest in your life and write it down in just one sentence. Visualize yourself receiving whatever it is that you want. Allow yourself to visualize every detail and get clear with it. Pay attention to how the halving of this thing makes you feel.

2. Once you have identified how the halving of this thing makes you feel, start creating this feeling place for yourself immediately. For example, if you visualized money because you want freedom or security, start finding ways to feel secure and free right now.

3. Keep your attention focused on that feeling place and then release and surrender to the Universe. Trust that your message has been delivered and that what you want is already there, you just need to open to it.

USE THIS PAGE TO MANIFEST:

_____
_____
_____
_____
_____
_____
_____
_____
_____
_____
_____
_____
_____
_____
_____
_____
_____
_____
_____
_____
_____
_____
_____
_____
_____
_____
_____
_____

Continue to Heal

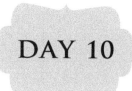

DAY 10

How was your day today?

_____

_____

_____

_____

_____

_____

_____

_____

_____

_____

_____

_____

_____

_____

_____

_____

_____

_____

_____

_____

_____

_____

_____

_____

_____

HOW CAN YOU HAVE A GREAT DAY TOMORROW?

You may say that is a hard question to answer but let's think how did you overcome yesterday?

- Did you speak with friends?

- Did you speak to your family?

- Did you think of happy thoughts?

- Did you do something that makes you happy?

- Do you have a hobby? If yes, what is it?

- Did you buy something that makes you smile?

_____

_____

_____

_____

_____

_____

_____

_____

_____

_____

_____

_____

_____

_____

Use this time to have the weekend for you....

- Play the video game

- Go to a spa

- Go on a date with yourself

- Go on a long ride

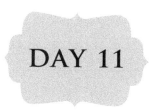

DAY 11

How was your day today?

_____
_____
_____
_____
_____
_____
_____
_____
_____
_____
_____
_____
_____
_____
_____
_____
_____
_____
_____
_____
_____
_____
_____
_____
_____
_____

HOW CAN YOU HAVE A GREAT DAY TOMORROW?

You may say that is a hard question to answer but let's think how did you overcome yesterday?

- Did you speak with friends?

- Did you speak to your family?

- Did you think of happy thoughts?

- Did you do something that makes you happy?

- Do you have a hobby? If yes, what is it?

- Did you buy something that makes you smile?

_____
_____
_____
_____
_____
_____
_____
_____
_____
_____
_____
_____
_____
_____

Exercise

- What is your deepest fear?

- Why does this scare you?

- What can you do to conquer that fear?

_____
_____
_____
_____
_____
_____
_____
_____
_____
_____
_____
_____
_____
_____
_____
_____
_____
_____
_____
_____
_____
_____
_____
_____

CONTINUED HERE.........

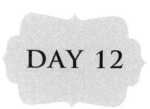

DAY 12

How was your day today?

_____
_____
_____
_____
_____
_____
_____
_____
_____
_____
_____
_____
_____
_____
_____
_____
_____
_____
_____
_____
_____
_____
_____
_____
_____
_____

HOW CAN YOU HAVE A GREAT DAY TOMORROW?

You may say that is a hard question to answer but let's think how did you overcome yesterday?

- Did you speak with friends?

- Did you speak to your family?

- Did you think of happy thoughts?

- Did you do something that makes you happy?

- Do you have a hobby? If yes, what is it?

- Did you buy something that makes you smile?

_____

_____

_____

_____

_____

_____

_____

_____

_____

_____

_____

_____

PRACTICE S.T.O.P.

Before school, during lunch, on your commute home, in the shower or before bed think to yourself, **S.T.O.P.**

S – Stop what you are doing for a minute.

T – Take a breath. Breathe normally and naturally and follow your breath coming in and of your nose.

O – Observe your thoughts. When a thought arises, acknowledge it, sit with it and accept it. Notice any emotions that are present and name them. Research indicates just naming your emotions can have a calming effect. Then focus on your body. Any physical sensations like a racing heart, tense muscles or pain? Identify it.

P – Proceed with something that will support you now. Whether that is talking to a friend or just stretching your shoulders.

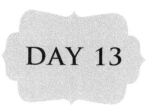

DAY 13

How was your day today?

_____

_____

_____

_____

_____

_____

_____

_____

_____

_____

_____

_____

_____

_____

_____

_____

_____

_____

_____

_____

_____

_____

_____

_____

_____

_____

HOW CAN YOU HAVE A GREAT DAY TOMORROW?

You may say that is a hard question to answer but let's think how did you overcome yesterday?

- Did you speak with friends?

- Did you speak to your family?

- Did you think of happy thoughts?

- Did you do something that makes you happy?

- Do you have a hobby? If yes, what is it?

- Did you buy something that makes you smile?

_____

_____

_____

_____

_____

_____

_____

_____

_____

_____

_____

_____

_____

_____

_____

If you are ever having bad thoughts just remember you are loved, you are cared for, you are the light of your parent's life. They want the best for you go talk to them and or go talk with a therapist. It is ok to reach out and get help from all over. Just go to a professional to talk through the things that may hunt you, that may taunt you, that may bother you.

HERE IS A LIST OF PROFESSIONALS:

National Suicide Prevention Lifeline
Call 1-800-273-8255

Youth Hotlines

The above crisis hotline is available for both adults and youths. If you're looking for a youth-specific line, you can try one of the following:

- Trevor Project Lifeline – Hotline for LGBT youth
  866-488-7386

- Child Help USA National Hotline – For youth who are suffering from child abuse
  1-800-4-A-CHILD (1-800-422-4453)

- Boys Town National Hotline – Serving all at-risk teens and children
  800-448-3000

- National Teen Dating Violence Hotline – Concerns about dating relationships
  1-866-331-9474 or text "loveis" to 22522

Sometimes life will kick you around, but sooner or later, you realize you're not just a survivor. You're a warrior, and you're stronger than anything life throws your way.

–Brooke Davis

CPSIA information can be obtained
at www.ICGtesting.com
Printed in the USA
LVHW042352170520
655882LV00002B/581